DAMIANA

A Comprehensive Guide to Cultivating,
Harvesting, and Harnessing the Aphrodisiac
Powers of Damiana..

Title:
DAMIANA

Subtitle

A Comprehensive Guide to Cultivating,
Harvesting, and Harnessing the Aphrodisiac
Powers of Damiana.

Copyright © 2024 by (Dr. Claud Treutel)

Printed in the United States of America.

ISBN: 9798880434824

TABLE OF CONTENT

INTRODUCTION

Few plants are as fascinating and alluring in the field of herbalism and natural treatments as Damiana (Turnera diffusa). Long regarded as a powerful aphrodisiac and adaptable medicinal plant, Damiana is indigenous to Central and South America and has been so for millennia. This thorough book takes us on a voyage to discover the delights of cultivating Damiana at home, as well as its rich history, needs for cultivation, and several health advantages, including its well-known aphrodisiac qualities.

What is Damiana?

Originally from Mexico, Texas, and portions of the Caribbean, Damiana, also known by its botanical name, Turnera diffusa, is a tiny shrub found in the subtropical areas of Central and South America. This fragrant plant, which belongs to the Turneraceae family, may reach a height of two meters and produces tiny, delicately scented yellow blooms.

Damiana has been used since prehistoric times when native Americans regarded it as a holy plant with a variety of ceremonial and medical uses. Damiana leaves were traditionally smoked or boiled into tea for their invigorating and uplifting properties. Damiana eventually spread beyond its homeland and became a staple in herbal treatment techniques all across the world.

Why Grow Damiana at Home?

There are several benefits to growing Damiana at home, which makes it a desirable option for both new and seasoned gardeners. The following are some strong arguments for thinking about growing Damiana in your garden:

- Accessibility: Damiana can easily be obtained by growing it at home, giving you direct access to fresh leaves that can be used right away in teas, tinctures, or culinary creations. However, it is also widely accessible as pills and herbal mixes.

- Quality Control: Since you are the one cultivating the plant, you can make sure that it is produced organically and picked at its greatest strength, which will maximize its medicinal advantages.

- Cost-Efficiency: Over time, buying Damiana pills or goods may prove to be costly. You may reap the advantages of Damiana without having to pay the recurrent expenses of purchasing it from the shop by growing your own.

Benefits of Damiana as an Aphrodisiac

Damiana is said to possess several qualities, but its reputation as a natural aphrodisiac is one of the most notable. For millennia, societies throughout have acknowledged and honored Damiana for its capacity to boost libido, increase sexual performance, and arouse desire. The following are the main advantages of Damiana as an aphrodisiac:

1. Enhanced Libido: Damiana is a well-liked option for people looking to improve their encounters because it is said to raise sexual desire and arousal in both men and women.

2. Better Sexual Performance: The chemicals in Damiana are believed to have a tonic impact on the reproductive system, which may help women lubricate their vaginas more effectively and improve erectile function in males.

3. Mood Enhancement: Damiana is well-known for its ability to uplift mood. This ability may help reduce tension, worry, and depression, which will make having sex more joyful and relaxed.

4. Enhanced Sensitivity: According to some anecdotal data, Damiana may enhance pleasure and sensory awareness within close

quarters, resulting in more satisfying sexual experiences.

5. Aphrodisiac Rituals: Damiana has been used in many cultural rituals and love traditions in addition to its physiological benefits.

GETTING STARTED WITH DAMIANA

Growing Damiana (Turnera diffusa) at home is a wonderful effort that opens the door to a world of herbalism, botanical inquiry, and self-sufficiency. If you are interested in learning more about these topics, you might consider beginning this adventure. In this part, we will go into the fundamental components of beginning to cultivate Damiana, beginning with a knowledge of the plant itself and moving on to selecting the appropriate environment and locating seeds or seedlings to get your garden off the ground.

Understanding Damiana Plant

Originally originating in the subtropical areas of Central and South America, the Damiana is a tiny shrub that is fragrant and belongs to the family of plants known as Turneraceae. It normally reaches a height of around two meters and is characterized by thin branches that are ornamented with leaves that are serrated and lance-shaped. Additionally, it yields exquisite yellow flowers that have a pleasant aroma.

The fragrant leaf of the Damiana plant, which, when crushed or damaged, gives off a pleasant, herbal odor, is one of the defining features of this plant. The leaves are the principal portion of the plant that is utilized for medical and culinary uses. They are highly appreciated for their alleged aphrodisiac qualities as well as their fragrant features.

When it comes to horticulture, Damiana is a plant that requires a modest amount of maintenance and thrives in soil that is well-drained and receives adequate sunlight to partial shade. Although it may thrive in a variety of soil types, it is most successful in sandy soil.

Climate and Growing Conditions

Damiana is indigenous to areas with subtropical temperatures, where it favors high levels of sunshine and warmth. Replicating these ideal circumstances is crucial when deciding where to grow Damiana indoors to promote strong growth and abundant flowering.

USDA hardiness zones 9–11 are the best places to grow Damiana since the temperatures there are continuously warm during the growing season. But in colder areas, Damiana may also be cultivated as an annual or container plant with the right maintenance and protection.

Damiana has a preference for temperatures between 70°F and 85°F (21°C to 29°C) during the day and above 60°F (15°C) at night. Damiana is susceptible to freezing temperatures, so keep it out of the cold and away from frost and extended periods.

Damiana does well in sunshine, ranging from full sun to moderate shade. For best development and flowering, try to get at least six hours of direct sunshine each day. Providing midday shade can assist avoid leaf blistering and keep soil moisture levels stable in areas with extreme heat.

For the cultivation of Damiana, drainage and soil quality are just as important as temperature and sunshine. Make sure the pH of the soil is between 5.5 and 6.5, slightly acidic, and well-drained. Adding organic materials to the soil, such as old manure or compost, can enhance its structure and fertility, encouraging strong root growth and general plant vigor.

Sourcing Damiana Seeds or Seedlings

Getting seeds or seedlings to start your garden is the next step after learning about the conditions for growing Damiana. Purchasing Damiana plants may be done in a few different ways, based on your preferences and availability:

1. Local Nurseries and Garden Centers: Find out whether the nurseries and garden centers in your region sell Damiana seedlings or seeds. Damiana is not as widely available as other herbs, although it may be found in specialist nurseries or those that sell medical plants.

2. Online Seed Providers: A large number of online seed providers provide a variety of herb seeds, including Damiana. Seek out trustworthy seed suppliers who have a history of producing high-quality seeds, good ratings, and a track record of doing so. Make sure the vendor ships to your location by checking their shipping policy before making an online purchase.

3. Wild Harvesting: You might be able to gather seeds or start new plants from existing stands if you reside in an area where Damiana grows naturally. But be careful while gathering wild food, and get the right licenses or authorization if needed. Make

sure you're not harming the natural environment or reducing wild population levels as well.

4. Seed Exchanges or Community Gardens: You might be able to swap Damiana seeds or cuttings with other enthusiasts by joining seed exchanges or community gardening clubs in your region. In addition, community gardens may offer a helpful setting where gardeners can exchange resources and expertise.

To ensure the highest chances of success, consider robust, healthy plants from reliable sources when choosing Damiana seeds or seedlings. If you are beginning from seeds, make sure you feed them enough warmth and moisture, then plant them according to the prescribed method. If you decide to go with seedlings, make sure they are planted in soil that has been prepared and give them constant attention to encourage development and establishment.

We will go into more depth about how to set up your Damiana garden in the following sections of this tutorial, including where to put your garden, how to prepare the soil, and how to sow seeds or seedlings. You may grow healthy Damiana plants at home if you have a good grasp of the plant's needs and take the right precautions.

SETTING UP YOUR DAMIANA GARDEN

The process of producing this fragrant and adaptable plant at home begins with the establishment of your Damiana garden, which is a key stage in the process. The success of your Damiana plants is dependent on several things, including the careful planting of the plants, the careful selection of the site, and the right preparation of the soil. Within the scope of this all-encompassing book, we will go into each of these facets in great detail, so equipping you with the information and direction you require to establish an optimum environment for the cultivation of Damiana.

Selecting the Right Location

When it comes to maintaining maximum development and output, selecting the appropriate site for your Damiana garden is of the utmost importance. To avoid waterlogging and root rot, Damiana has to be grown in soil that has good drainage. It would also benefit from warm, sunny circumstances. Concerning the selection of a place for your Damiana garden, the following are some factors to take into consideration:

- Sunshine: Damiana needs lots of sunlight to grow well. Select a spot that gets six to eight hours of direct sunshine each day. The best locations are those that face south or west as they usually get the most sunshine during the day.

- Wind Protection: Damianas can withstand a certain amount of wind exposure, but strong winds can harm the delicate blooms and leaves. If at all feasible, locate yourself somewhere with some wind shelter, such as next to a structure, hedge, or fence.

- Temperature: Damiana is susceptible to frost and does best in warm climates. Choose a spot where the weather is continuously warm during the growth season; stay away from regions that are vulnerable to chilly winds or frost pockets.

- Accessibility: Take into account how easy it will be to irrigate, harvest, and maintain the chosen area. For frequent maintenance and attention, the garden should ideally be conveniently accessible from your house or garden shed.

- Room Availability: Determine how much space your garden has to provide and make plans appropriately. Because dahlia plants spread out as they grow, make sure there is adequate space for them to do so without crowding out other plants or buildings.

By giving careful consideration to these aspects, you will be able to choose a place that offers the optimal growing circumstances for your Damiana plants, therefore laying the groundwork for a big harvest.

Soil Preparation and Requirements

To build a Damiana garden that is both healthy and fruitful, one of the most important steps is to prepare the soil. Soil that is well-drained, rich in nutrients, and has a somewhat acidic pH level is ideal for the growth of Damiana. For your Damiana plants, the following is a guide on how to prepare the soil:

- Soil Testing: To determine the pH and nutritional content of your soil, test it before planting. The ideal pH range for Damiana is between 5.5 and 6.5. To get the ideal pH level for Damiana cultivation, amend the soil as necessary.

- Enhancing Drainage: If the soil gets wet, Damiana is vulnerable to root rot. By adding organic matter to the soil, such as compost or well-rotted manure, you may guarantee adequate drainage. This will supply vital nutrients for plant growth and aid in enhancing the drainage and structure of the soil.

- Adding Amendments: To address nutrient imbalances or deficiencies, add any amendments that are required based on the findings of your soil test. Greensand (for potassium), sulfur, and bone meal (for phosphorus) are common soil additions used in Damiana cultivation (for lowering pH).

- Tilling the Soil: Till the soil to a depth of eight to ten inches with a garden fork or tiller. In addition to aerating the soil, this will make it friable and loose, which will encourage root penetration and development.

- Mulching: After planting Damiana, think about covering the soil's surface with a layer of organic mulch, such as wood chips or straw. Mulch creates an environment that is ideal for plant growth by regulating soil temperature, preventing weed growth, and assisting in the retention of soil moisture.

By devoting some of your time to the process of correctly preparing the soil, you can provide your Damiana plants with the ideal growth environment, hence increasing the likelihood that they will flourish in your garden.

Planting Damiana: Step-by-Step Guide

When you have chosen the ideal spot and made the necessary preparations for the soil, it is time to plant your Damiana seeds or seedlings. You ensure that the planting procedure goes smoothly, be sure to follow these detailed directions with each step:

Prepare Planting Holes: Dig planting holes that are a little bit deeper and broader than the seedling's root ball if you're planting Damiana seedlings. To ensure that there is sufficient space between plants, plant holes should be spaced at least 12 to 18 inches apart.

Transplant Seedlings: Take the Damiana seedlings out of their pots with caution, and then gently pull apart any knotted roots. Make sure the top of the root ball of each seedling is level with the surrounding soil surface by placing it into a planting hole.

Backfill Soil: To guarantee proper soil-to-root contact, fill up the planting holes with soil and gently push down around the base of each seedling. To eliminate any air pockets around the roots and settle the soil, give the area a thorough watering.

Watering: To promote root establishment, give the Damiana seedlings a thorough irrigation after planting. During the first establishing phase, keep the soil continuously damp but not soggy. After the plants are well-established, progressively cut back on the number of waterings, letting the soil somewhat dry out in between.

Mulching: To help keep the soil wet and prevent weed growth, add a layer of organic mulch around the base of the Damiana plants. To avoid moisture-related problems and deter pests, leave a tiny space between the mulch and the plant stems.

Maintenance: Keep a constant eye out for growth and health indicators on your Damiana plants. Get rid of any weeds that could be in the way of the plant's need for water and nutrients. If required, provide support for the plants as they grow, such as cages or stakes.

If you follow these instructions, you will be able to plant your Damiana seedlings with complete assurance, putting them on the way to robust development and plentiful harvests.

CARING FOR YOUR DAMIANA PLANTS

Providing proper care for your Damiana plants is necessary to guarantee their well-being, vigor, and output. To properly care for Damianas, it is necessary to pay attention to the following critical components during the growth season: watering, fertilizer, and pest management strategies. We are going to go into each of these factors in this detailed guide, which will provide you with the knowledge and guidance you need to efficiently care for your Damiana plants.

Watering Schedule

Because both insufficient and excessive moisture can have an impact on the growth and health of plants, watering is an essential component of Damiana's care. Once established, Damiana plants can tolerate drought conditions, even though they prefer evenly moist soil. To create a watering regimen for your Damiana plants, the following rules should be followed:

- Establishment Period: To promote root development, give Damiana seedlings plenty of water during the first several days following planting. Maintain a constant moisture content in the soil, but do not let it become too wet—let extra water evaporate naturally.

- Water your Damiana plants frequently, especially in the summer when the weather is hot and dry. Depending on the weather and soil moisture levels, try to water deeply once or twice a week. Using your finger to probe the soil around the plant bases, determine the moisture content of the soil frequently. When the top inch of soil appears dry to the touch, add water.

- Watering in the morning: Give Damiana plants a morning watering to reduce evaporation and give the leaves time to dry before dusk. Overnight wet foliage might make fungal infections more likely.

- Steer clear of overwatering: Damiana plants are prone to root rot if the soil is wet for a long time. Let the soil dry out a little bit in between waterings to prevent overwatering. Don't grow Damiana in poorly drained regions; instead, use a soil mixture that drains well.

- Mulching: To assist conserve soil moisture and controlling soil temperature, use an organic mulch layer around the base of Damiana plants. Mulch also lessens competition for water and nutrients by inhibiting the development of weeds.

You can guarantee that your Damiana plants receive the moisture they require to flourish without succumbing to water-related concerns if you adhere to a consistent watering schedule and check the levels of moisture in the soil.

Fertilization Tips

It is vital to fertilize Damiana plants appropriately to provide them with the nutrients that they require to encourage healthy growth and development. It is possible to improve growth and output by fertilizing Damiana on occasion, even though it requires very little maintenance in comparison to other plants. A few pointers to consider when fertilizing your Damiana plants are as follows:

- Timing: Early spring is the best time to fertilize Damiana plants, right before new growth appears. This gives the plant an extra nutritional boost to encourage blooming and rapid development all through the growing season.

- Use a water-soluble fertilizer that is balanced and has equal amounts of potassium, phosphorus, and nitrogen (N-P-K). Alternatively, since Damiana has tiny yellow flowers, you may use a fertilizer made especially for plants that bloom.

- Application Method: Apply the fertilizer to the soil surrounding the base of Damiana plants after diluting it according to the manufacturer's recommendations. Fertilizer should not be applied straight to the foliage as this might burn the leaves.

- During the growth season, fertilize Damiana plants every four to six weeks; when the plants go dormant in late autumn or winter, fertilization should be sporadic. Steer clear of overfertilizing as this might result in luxuriant foliage at the price of flower output.

- Organic Options: You may fertilize Damiana plants using compost or well-rotted manure if you'd rather follow an organic gardening schedule. In spring, cover the base of the plants with a thin layer of manure or compost. This will help retain moisture and keep weeds at bay. Next, cover the mulch layer over the compost.

It is possible to encourage strong development and ensure abundant flowering throughout the growing season by giving Damiana plants the appropriate balance of nutrients through the

application of appropriate fertilizer.

Pest and Disease Management

Even though Damiana is highly resistant to illnesses and pests, there are still certain problems that may occur on occasion and require treatment. For your convenience, the following is a list of common diseases and pests that can harm Damiana plants, as well as some tactics for managing them:

- Aphids: Damiana plants can become infested by these tiny, sap-sucking insects, which result in stunted growth and deformed leaves. Aphids can be removed from plants by spraying them with a powerful stream of water, or as a natural substitute, by applying neem oil or insecticidal soap.

- Spider mites: Spider mites are microscopic arachnids that cause stippled or fading leaves by feeding on the sap of Damiana plants. Spraying plants with water frequently can help reduce dust and boost humidity, both of which will help keep spider mites at bay. Use a horticultural oil or insecticidal soap to treat the afflicted plants if the infestation is severe.

- Powdery Mildew: Powdery mildew is a fungal disease that can inflict white, powdery areas on the leaves of Damiana plants. Make sure there is adequate air circulation around Damiana plants by appropriately spacing them apart and avoiding overcrowding to prevent powdery mildew. If powdery mildew appears, use a fungicidal spray containing potassium bicarbonate or sulfur on the afflicted plants.

- Root Rot: Damiana plants cultivated in very wet or poorly drained soil may develop root rot, a fungal disease. Make sure the soil is well-drained and refrain from overwatering to prevent root rot. Remove impacted plants and enhance soil drainage if root rot is detected to stop the illness from spreading.

- Leaf Miners: Leaf miners are tiny larvae that burrow into Damiana plant leaves, leaving behind blotches or trails that are ugly. Use insecticidal soap or neem oil to treat afflicted plants, or remove and destroy diseased leaves to control leaf miners.

You can ensure that your Damiana plants remain healthy and flourishing throughout the growing season by adhering to proper garden hygiene practices, keeping a close eye on the plants to identify any symptoms of pests or illnesses, and taking early action to treat any problems that may occur.

HARVESTING AND PRESERVING DAMIANA

The cultivation of this multipurpose herb begins with the harvesting and preservation of Damiana, which is an essential stage in the process. When you utilize Damiana leaves in teas, tinctures, and culinary creations, it is important to ensure that you catch the most amount of their potency and flavor by using the appropriate timing and procedures. In this all-encompassing tutorial, we will discuss every facet of harvesting and preserving Damiana, including the knowledge of when to harvest, the methods of harvesting, as well as the drying and storing of Damiana leaves for long-term usage.

Knowing When to Harvest

It is crucial to determine the best moment to harvest Damiana leaves to capture the most flavor and power of these delicate leaves. It is possible to collect Damiana leaves at any point throughout the growing season; however, the timing of harvesting may vary based on the purpose of the leaves and your personal preferences. When it comes to knowing when to harvest Damiana, here are some rules to follow:

• Leaf Development: When daisy leaves achieve full maturity and take on a deep green hue, they are usually ready for harvesting. Small or undeveloped leaves should not be harvested since they may not have the full flavor and scent of mature leaves.

- Blooming Stage: During the growth season, dahiana plants have the potential to produce tiny, yellow blooms. Although the blossoms are not usually taken, their appearance might indicate that the plant is about ready to be harvested. To preserve the maximum flavor and strength of the Damiana leaves, harvest them before the blossoms fully open.

- Look for evidence of maturity in the look of the Damiana leaves. When leaves reach maturity, they are glossy, firm, and devoid of defects or discoloration. Steer clear of picking leaves that exhibit symptoms of illness, injury, or insect infestation.

- Time of Day: Harvest Damiana departs early in the morning, just as the dew starts to disappear but before the temperature rises. Harvesting in the morning ensures a higher-quality crop by preserving the taste and essential oils in the leaves.

- Harvesting Damiana leaves regularly will help to promote growth and productivity throughout the growing season. Removing all of a plant's leaves at once should be avoided since this may cause stress and stunt the plant's ability to thrive in the future.

It is possible to guarantee that you harvest Damiana leaves at their best flavor and potency by paying attention to these markers. This will allow you to make the most of the culinary and medical benefits that these leaves provide.

Harvesting Techniques

After you have established that the leaves of your Damiana plant are sufficiently mature to be harvested, it is time to collect them from the plant. The following is a list of methods that may be utilized to harvest Damiana:

1. Handpicking: This is the most popular way of gathering Damiana leaves. Mature leaves should be carefully removed from the stems, being careful not to harm the nearby flowers or foliage. With a small section of the stem left intact, carefully cut the leaves off the plant with sharp scissors or pruning shears.

2. Selective Harvesting: Remove only the mature leaves from a plant as needed, as opposed to gathering all of the leaves from it at once. This makes it possible for the plant to keep growing throughout the growing season, guaranteeing a steady supply of newly harvested leaves.

3. Preventing Overharvesting: Damiana plants are hardy and tolerant of light pruning, but to prevent overharvesting, leave enough foliage on the plant to sustain its health and growth. At each harvest, try to harvest no more than one-third of the total leaf mass from a single plant.

4. Gentle Handling: Take caution when handling harvested Damiana leaves to avoid cuts or damage. To absorb excess moisture and shield the leaves from damage during transit, place them in a clean basket or container lined with paper towels.

5. Gathering Flowers and Stems: Damiana plants can yield flowers and stems that can be collected for usage in herbal remedies, in addition to their leaves. To enjoy the fullest flavor and aroma, harvest flowers before they fully open. Trim stems as needed to allow air to circulate and avoid crowding.

You can harvest Damiana leaves and other plant parts with minimal damage by using these harvesting techniques, which will guarantee a high-quality harvest for both culinary and medicinal uses.

Drying and Storing Damiana

Once the Damiana leaves have been picked, they must be dried and stored appropriately to maintain their flavor, aroma, and therapeutic benefits. For long-term usage, the following is a guide on how to dry and preserve Damiana leaves:

- Air Drying: Air drying is the most popular technique for preserving Damiana leaves. Arrange the gathered leaves in a single layer on a sanitized, dehydrated surface, like a baking sheet or wire rack. Make sure there is enough airflow around the leaves and that they are not touching.

- Location for Drying: To dry Damiana leaves, pick an area with good ventilation, low humidity, and indirect sunshine. The leaves may lose flavor and color if they are dried in direct sunlight.

- Drying Time: Depending on the climate and leaf thickness, damana leaves normally take one to two weeks to dry entirely. Regularly check the leaves for dryness, and remove any that seem brittle and crispy to the touch.

- Other Drying Methods: If you'd like, you may also use a low-temperature oven or dehydrator to dry Damiana leaves (around 100°F to 120°F). Arrange the leaves in a solitary layer on a baking sheet or drying tray and allow them to dry until they become fragile and crunchy.

- Storage Jars: After the leaves have dried, place them in fresh, airtight jars or plastic bags that can be sealed. Put the harvest date on the containers' labels, then keep them out of direct sunlight and moisture in a cool, dark spot.

- Shelf Life: Damiana leaves can keep their flavor and potency for up to a year or more if they are dried and stored properly. Periodically inspect the leaves for evidence of moisture or mildew, and dispose of those that appear to be deteriorating.

The flavor, fragrance, and medicinal benefits of Damiana leaves may be preserved for long-term usage in teas, tinctures, and culinary creations if you follow these drying and storage processes by following the instructions.

UTILIZING DAMIANA IN CULINARY DELIGHTS

Damiana is a great addition to a variety of culinary preparations because of its distinct taste profile and fragrant properties. With a hint of herbal refinement, Damiana adds its essence to enrich foods and beverages, from tasty cocktails and sumptuous sweets to calming teas. This extensive tutorial will go over several ways to use Damiana in food preparation, such as diverse tea recipes, inventive cocktail and dessert ideas, and unique cooking methods to infuse meals with Damiana flavor.

Different Recipes for Damiana Tea

Damiana tea is a traditional method of indulging in the herbal essence of this adaptable plant. It is highly regarded for its calming qualities and delicate floral overtones. Damiana tea provides both comfort and vitality, whether savored unadulterated or combined with other herbs and spices. Here are some recipes to try for Damiana tea:

- Traditional Damiana Tea: Steep dried Damiana leaves in boiling water for five to ten minutes, then drain and drink. To add a hint of sweetness or acidity, taste and add honey or lemon.

- Damiana Mint Tea: For a revitalizing take on the classic Damiana tea, mix dried Damiana leaves with fresh mint leaves. For a fragrant, minty tea that calms the senses and promotes digestion, steep the leaves in hot water together.

- Damiana Chai Tea: To make a spiced variant of Damiana tea, steep dried Damiana leaves with cardamom, cloves, ginger, and cinnamon. For a decadent and rich dessert, add milk and sugar to taste.

- Damiana Citrus Tea: Add the vibrant tastes of citrus fruits, including orange, lemon, or grapefruit, to Damiana tea. When the tea is steeping, add slices or zest of citrus to give it a cool, refreshing taste.

- Damiana Iced Tea: Brew Damiana tea according to the recipe, then let it cool in the fridge. For a cool summertime drink, serve over ice with a slice of lemon or a sprig of fresh mint.

Create your own special Damiana tea variants by experimenting with different herbal combinations and flavor profiles that suit your mood and taste preferences.

Incorporating Damiana in Cocktails and Desserts

Beyond tea, Damiana infuses drinks and pastries with its unique herbal flavor and fragrant scent, giving them depth and complexity. Here are some inventive ways to use Damiana in your culinary creations, ranging from tasty drinks to rich desserts:

- Damiana Margarita: For a Mexican-inspired take on the traditional margarita, mix Damiana liqueur with tequila, triple sec, and fresh lime juice. Serve this fragrant and delicious drink over ice with a salted rim.

- Damiana Mojito: Muddle fresh mint leaves with simple syrup and lime wedges, then stir in white rum and Damiana liqueur. For a cool and herbal mojito, add club soda on top and garnish with a mint leaf.

- Damiana Old Fashioned: Combine Damiana liqueur with rye or bourbon whiskey, a sugar cube, and a splash of bitters. Serve over ice with an orange peel twist for a chic and fragrant spin on the traditional Old Fashioned drink.

- Damiana Chocolate Truffles: After gently heating heavy cream, soak Damiana leaves in it for ten to fifteen minutes. After straining the cream, use it to make truffle chocolate ganache. For a decadent treat, roll the truffles in chopped almonds or chocolate powder.

- Damiana Panna Cotta: Use Damiana leaves to infuse milk or cream, and then use the resulting mixture to make a traditional panna cotta flavored with honey and vanilla. Serve this lovely and light dessert with a sprinkle of honey or fresh fruit.

Try your hand at several desserts and drink recipes to find fresh and interesting ways to use Damiana in your cooking.

Cooking with Damiana: Creative Ideas

Damiana's herbal essence and fragrant properties may be utilized to flavor savory foods as well as drinks and sweets. Here are some imaginative mealtime suggestions for Damiana:

- Damiana-infused Oil or Vinegar: Soak dried Damiana leaves in olive oil or vinegar to make a tasty infusion for salads, marinades, or sauces. Use the infused oil or vinegar to give a mild herbal flavor to grilled veggies, shellfish, and roasted meats.

- Damiana Risotto: For a mild herbal taste and aromatic richness, stir dried Damiana leaves into a standard risotto dish. Stir the leaves and broth into the risotto, allowing them to permeate the dish with their flavor while it cooks.

- Damiana Scented Rice: To make a fragrant and aromatic side dish, steep dry Damiana leaves in water before cooking rice with infused water. Serve the Damiana-scented rice with grilled fish or chicken for a tasty and beautiful supper.

- Damiana-infused Syrup: To make a simple syrup, heat water, sugar, and dried Damiana leaves together until the sugar dissolves. The syrup may be used to sweeten cocktails, lemonade, or iced tea, or drizzled over pancakes or waffles to create a distinctive and tasty topping.

- Damiana-infused Sauce: For an unexpected taste boost, mix dried Damiana leaves into a prepared sauce or gravy. Simmer the leaves with tomatoes, onions, garlic, and herbs to make a flavorful sauce that goes well with pasta, meat, and vegetables.

Get creative in the kitchen and try new ways to include Damiana in your favorite dishes. Damiana, whether used in drinks, sweets, or savory meals, lends a distinct and unforgettable flavor to culinary creations, enhancing them with its herbal essence and olfactory appeal.

EXPLORING DAMIANA'S APHRODISIAC PROPERTIES

The Damiana, a little shrub that is indigenous to the subtropical parts of Central and South America, has been respected for a very long time due to the aphrodisiac powers that it is said to possess. Throughout human history, Damiana has been lauded for its capacity to increase desire, stimulate sexual energy, and foster connection. During this in-depth investigation, we will investigate the historical and cultural significance of Damiana, investigate the effects that it has on libido, and investigate the innovative ways that Damiana may be used in loving rituals.

Historical and Cultural Significance

For millennia, Damiana (Turnera diffusa) has been used as a tonic and aphrodisiac plant. Native American groups from Central and South America, such as the Aztecs and Mayans, held Damiana in high regard due to its therapeutic qualities and ceremonial importance. Traditionally, the leaves of the Damiana plant were smoked or made into teas to enhance mood and libido.

Damiana was revered as a sacred herb by the ancient Aztecs and was connected to Xochiquetzal, the fertility and love goddess. It was frequently a part of sacrifices and ceremonies honoring romance, love, and fertility. In a similar vein, the Mayans believed Damiana to be a strong aphrodisiac that could improve relationships and foster marital joy, thus they employed it in ceremonies to increase sexual desire and pleasure.

Later, after traveling across the Americas, European explorers and settlers came across Damiana and brought back stories of its aphrodisiac qualities. Damiana was incorporated into traditional herbal medicine techniques when it became well-known in Europe as a natural treatment for low libido and sexual dysfunction.

Damiana is still valued for its capacity to improve intimacy and sexual vigor and is still renowned for its aphrodisiac qualities. It is still regarded as essential to herbal medicine traditions worldwide because of its all-encompassing approach to promoting sexual health and well-being.

Understanding Damiana's Effects on Libido

The complex combination of bioactive substances found in Damiana, such as flavonoids, terpenoids, and essential oils, is thought to have aphrodisiac qualities. These substances are believed to have a variety of physiological benefits, such as improving mood, boosting circulation, and encouraging relaxation, all of which may lead to an increase in libido and sexual desire.

- Increasing Circulation: Damiana is said to possess vasodilatory properties, which entail the ability to enlarge blood vessels and enhance blood flow to all parts of the body, including the vaginal area. A more enjoyable sexual encounter might result from increased sensitivity and excitement brought on by improved circulation.

- Mood Enhancement: Damiana includes ingredients that may have a slight sedative effect, bringing on sensations of bliss, contentment, and relaxation. Damiana can improve general sexual satisfaction and foster an intimate atmosphere by lowering tension and anxiety.

- Increasing Vitality and Energy: Damiana's supporters think that it has a natural energy-boosting effect that makes people feel more energized and vigorous. Increased stamina and performance in the bedroom may result from this, enabling longer and more fulfilling sex sessions.

- Hormone Balancing: Damiana may have a balancing impact on hormone levels, namely those of estrogen and testosterone. Damiana may assist both men and women with symptoms of hormonal imbalances, including reduced libido, by regulating hormone levels.

Although there is no scientific study on Damiana's aphrodisiac qualities, historical tales and anecdotal data point to possible benefits for libido and sexual function. After using Damiana, many people claim to have greater sexual pleasure, heightened arousal, and increased sensitivity.

Incorporating Damiana into Romantic Rituals

Damiana is a perfect addition to love rituals and to improve intimate times with a partner because of its sensuous perfume and aphrodisiac properties. Damiana may set the mood for romance and create a special shared experience, whether it's in the shape of a rich dessert, a fragrant tea, or an opulent massage oil. Here are some inventive methods to include Damiana in romantic customs:

Damiana Tea Ceremony: Make a pot of Damiana tea, then spend some time in silence enjoying the aromatic infusion and its calming properties. To add intimacy and sweetness, squeeze in a little lemon or honey.

Damiana-infused Bath: Infuse a warm bath with bath oils or salts to create a romantic ambiance. A wonderful evening together will be created by the body-calming waters and fragrant steam, which will also arouse the senses.

Damiana Massage Oil: To make a posh massage oil, mix Damiana essential oil with carrier oil, like sweet almond or jojoba oil. For a wonderfully calming and sensuous experience, massage your partner's body with soft, rhythmic strokes, paying particular attention to sensitive and tense regions.

Damiana-infused Cuisine: Use Damiana as a seasoning for savory or dessert dishes to add a romantic touch to your dinner menu. From rich chocolate truffles to marinades and sauces enhanced with Damiana, express your culinary creativity while you entice your palate and delight your senses in tandem.

Damiana Aromatherapy: To improve closeness and create a romantic atmosphere, diffuse Damiana essential oil in the bedroom. Damiana's warm, woodsy scent can enhance arousal and relaxation, stimulating the senses and strengthening bonds between lovers.

Couples may build deeper ties and increase the joy of being together by introducing Damiana to love rituals and shared experiences. This will produce important moments of connection and intimacy.

POTENTIAL RISKS AND PRECAUTIONS

Even though most people consider Damiana to be safe when used moderately, it's important to be aware of any potential hazards and take appropriate care when using it. Damiana, like any herbal medicine, has the potential to combine with drugs, have negative effects, or be dangerous for certain people. This thorough guide will go over the possible hazards and safety measures associated with taking Damiana, such as adverse reactions and side effects, interactions with drugs, and safe intake guidelines.

Side Effects and Allergic Reactions

When taken properly, Damiana is thought to be safe for the majority of people, yet some people may have allergic responses or have negative effects. The following are typical adverse effects of Damiana consumption:

Gastrointestinal Disturbances: After using Damiana, some people may have gastrointestinal symptoms such as nausea, vomiting, or diarrhea. Although these symptoms are usually mild and temporary, some people may find them unpleasant.

Headache: Damiana consumption has the potential to sometimes cause headaches or migraines, especially in people who are hormonally sensitive or have a history of headaches.

Allergic Reactions: In rare cases, people may develop an allergic response to Damiana, which is characterized by symptoms including breathing difficulties, hives, rash, itching, and swelling of the face or throat. If, after taking Damiana, you notice any symptoms of an allergic reaction, get medical help right once.

Hormonal Effects: Damiana may alter the body's levels of testosterone and estrogen. Mild hormonal effects have also been recorded. Before using Damiana, anyone with hormone-sensitive illnesses including prostate cancer, uterine fibroids, or breast cancer should exercise caution and speak with a healthcare professional.

Pregnancy and Nursing: The safety of Damiana during pregnancy and breastfeeding is not well understood. Damiana has long been used to promote reproductive health, but little research has been done on whether it is safe to take during pregnancy or breastfeeding. Damiana should not be taken by pregnant or nursing mothers unless specifically instructed by a healthcare professional.

It's critical to keep an eye on how Damiana affects your body and to stop using it if you feel uncomfortable or have any negative side effects. Before using Damiana, see a trained healthcare provider if you have any underlying medical issues or are concerned about any possible adverse effects.

Interactions with Medications

Damiana may interact with other medicines, thereby compromising the safety or effectiveness of such drugs. Damiana should be used with caution if you are taking any drugs, especially those that have been known to interact with herbs or supplements. The following are a few examples of drugs that Damiana may interact with:

- Anticoagulant Drugs: Damiana may have minor blood-thinning (anticoagulant) effects. These effects may interact with anticoagulant drugs such as aspirin or warfarin (Coumadin). Damiana and some drugs together may make bleeding or bruises more likely.

- Diabetes Medication: Damiana has the potential to reduce blood sugar levels, which might cause interactions with oral hypoglycemic drugs or insulin, two common diabetes treatments. If you are using Damiana together with diabetic medication, keep a close eye on your blood sugar levels and change the amount of your medication as necessary under the supervision of a healthcare professional.

- Medication for Sedation: Damiana has a small amount of sedative or central nervous system depressant effects, which means that it may intensify the effects of benzodiazepines or barbiturates, among other prescriptions. Damiana and some drugs together may make you feel more sleepy or lightheaded.

- Hormone Replacement Therapy (HRT): Damiana may interact with hormone replacement therapy (HRT) drugs and have hormonal effects of her own. When using Damiana, those on HRT should exercise caution and speak with a healthcare professional first.

- Contraceptive Drugs: Damiana may have modest hormonal side effects and may reduce the effectiveness of birth control pills and other contraceptive drugs. Before using Damiana, women who use hormonal contraception should speak with a healthcare professional.

It's crucial to go over Damiana's possible side effects and interactions with your doctor before using it if you take any drugs. Considering your unique health situation and prescribed drug schedule, your healthcare practitioner can assist you in deciding if Damiana is safe and suitable for you.

Safety Guidelines for Consumption

To minimize the danger of unwanted effects and ensure that Damiana is consumed safely, the following safety considerations should be considered:

Beginning with a Low Dose: If you are unfamiliar with Damiana or unsure about the impact it will have on your body, it is recommended that you begin with a low dose and gradually raise it as required. As a result, you will be able to evaluate how your body reacts and reduce the likelihood of experiencing any negative consequences.

Pay Attention to Side Effects: It is important to pay attention to how your body reacts to Damiana and to keep an eye out for any symptoms of uncomfortable side effects or allergic responses. If you have any unpleasant effects, such as nausea, rash, or trouble breathing, you should immediately stop using the product and seek medical treatment.

Contact a Healthcare Practitioner Before using Damiana, it is important to consult with a trained healthcare provider if you have any preexisting health issues, are currently taking any drugs, or have any questions regarding the overall safety of the product. Your healthcare practitioner can offer you individualized assistance and assist you in determining whether or not Damiana is suitable for you and secure for your needs.

To reduce the likelihood of experiencing negative effects, it is important to use Damiana in a responsible manner and moderation. If you have preexisting health concerns or are at risk for unpleasant reactions, you should avoid using the product for an extended period or in excessive amounts.

Invest in Products of Superior Quality: To guarantee that your Damiana is both pure and effective, choose goods of excellent quality that come from trusted suppliers. You should look for items that have been evaluated by independent third-party laboratories to determine their level of quality and safety.

With the help of these safety precautions and the exercise of caution when taking Damiana, you will be able to reduce the likelihood of experiencing any negative effects and confidently take advantage of any possible advantages it may provide.

BEYOND THE BASICS: ADVANCED TIPS AND TECHNIQUES

As you become more experienced with growing Damiana, investigating more sophisticated methods and strategies will enable you to maximize your yield and realize the full potential of this adaptable plant. There are plenty of options to investigate on your trip with Damiana, from perfecting propagation techniques to optimizing production and experimenting with various types. We will explore advanced cultivation tips and practices for Damiana in this extensive tutorial, covering how to propagate your plants, how to maximize production, and how to experiment with different types to improve your growing experience.

Propagation Methods

The act of creating new Damiana plants from seed or cuttings taken from an existing plant is known as propagation. Damiana is mostly cultivated from seeds, but you may increase the size of your Damiana garden by using different propagation techniques to create new plants. Consider these cutting-edge propagation techniques:

1. Seed Propagation: Using seeds is the most popular way to spread Damiana. Gather seed from established Damiana plants and plant it in a well-draining soil mixture, softly covering the seed with earth. It should take two to four weeks for germination to occur if

the soil is kept warm and constantly wet. After seedlings have produced multiple sets of true leaves, transplant them into separate pots.

2. Cutting Propagation: Although less frequently used than seed propagation, damana may also be produced from stem cuttings. Ensure that the cuttings you take from well-established, robust Damiana plants have several nodes throughout the stem. To promote the growth of roots, remove any lower leaves from the cutting and immerse the cut end in the rooting hormone. Once the cutting is planted, place

it in a soil mixture that drains well and keep it constantly wet until roots form.

3. Division: Dividing mature plants into smaller portions and replanting them is another way of Damiana propagation. A mature Damiana plant's root ball should be carefully dug out and divided into smaller portions, ensuring that each section includes both roots and shoots. Replant the separated pieces, keeping the soil wet until new growth appears, either directly in the garden or in individual containers.

You may easily propagate new plants and grow your Damiana garden by learning these sophisticated propagation techniques.

Maximizing Damiana Yield

It's crucial to provide your Damiana plants with the best-growing conditions and maintenance during the growing season if you want to optimize their production and productivity. The following advanced advice can help you maximize Damiana's yield:

- Ideal Growing Conditions: Damiana grows best in warm, sunny spots with sufficient air circulation and soil that drains well. To increase fertility and drainage, select a location that receives full sun exposure and enrich the soil with organic materials like compost or aged manure.

- Frequent Care: Watering, fertilizing, and controlling pests are all part of regular care that will keep Damiana plants robust and healthy. Regularly check plants for symptoms of pests, illnesses, or nutrient shortages, and respond quickly to any problems that are discovered.

- Training & Pruning: By eliminating damaged or dead foliage and promoting the growth of new branches, pruning Damiana plants can assist in encouraging bushy growth and enhance output. Regularly pinching back the ends of stems will train plants to grow compact and upright.

- When to Harvest: Damiana leaves should be harvested in late summer or early fall, when they are completely developed and scented. With a little section of the stem left intact, carefully cut the leaves off the plant with sharp scissors or pruning shears. By keeping enough leaves on the plant to maintain its development and health, you may prevent overharvesting.

- Crop Rotation: To avoid soil erosion and reduce the accumulation of pests and illnesses, alternate your Damiana plants with other crops in your garden. To keep soil fertility and balance, alternate Damiana with heavy feeders like tomatoes squash, or legumes that fix nitrogen.

You may increase the fertility and yield of your Damiana garden and guarantee a plentiful harvest of fragrant foliage for both culinary and medicinal purposes by putting these sophisticated suggestions and procedures into practice.

Experimenting with Different Varieties

Other species and variations of Turnera offer distinctive flavors and qualities, while Damiana (Turnera diffusa) is the most widely grown variant used for its therapeutic and aphrodisiac qualities. Try experimenting with different Damiana kinds to spice up your garden and broaden your culinary and medicinal horizons. Consider the following several Damiana varieties:

Turnera ulmifolia: Often referred to as false Damiana or ramgoat dash along, this closely related plant is occasionally confused with Damiana. It may have somewhat distinct flavor characteristics, but it has comparable fragrant leaves and yellow blooms.

Turnera diffusa var. aphrodisiaca: This Damiana variation is grown especially for its strong flavor and scent, which are said to have aphrodisiac qualities. It is frequently utilized in aphrodisiac and herbal remedy formulations.

Turnera subulata: Another species of Turnera with fragrant leaves and little white blooms, often called white alder. It shares a similar flavor characteristic with Damiana, although being less often utilized. It may be used for both medical and culinary purposes.

Hybrid Kinds: To produce new cultivars with distinctive qualities, several farmers have experimented with crossing different Damiana varieties. These hybrid species have fascinating opportunities for culinary and therapeutic applications, as they may display variances in flavor, scent, and growing patterns.

Experimenting with several Damiana kinds can reveal the diversity of this adaptable plant and stimulate the development of new gastronomic and therapeutic products. There are many possibilities to fit every taste and inclination, whether you're interested in trying out unusual hybrids or conventional Damiana species.

FREQUENTLY ASKED QUESTIONS (FAQS)

As the number of people interested in cultivating and making use of Damiana continues to increase, it is only inevitable that concerns will arise concerning its cultivation, applications, and effects. In this extensive guide, we will address some of the most commonly asked questions (FAQs) regarding Damiana. These questions will include typical inquiries about cultivating Damiana as well as concerns about the aphrodisiac properties of the plant.

Common Queries about Growing Damiana

Which climate is ideal for Damiana cultivation?

Warm, subtropical regions with lots of sunshine and soil that drains well are ideal for Damiana growth. USDA zones 9 through 11 allow outdoor growing, whereas colder areas require container gardening.

What is the duration required for Damiana seeds to sprout?

Under ideal circumstances, damana seeds usually germinate in two to four weeks. To promote germination, maintain the soil's constant moisture content and warmth.

How often should I water my Damiana plants?

Damiana plants need regular irrigation, especially in hot, dry weather, and appreciate slightly damp soil. Steer clear of overwatering Damiana since soggy soil might lead to root rot.

What time of year is ideal for harvesting Damiana leaves?

Although damana leaves can be collected at any point throughout the growing season, it is ideal to do it in late summer or early fall, when the leaves are fully developed and fragrant.

Can one grow Damiana indoors?

It is possible to cultivate Damiana indoors in containers with the right ventilation and illumination. To ensure that there is enough light for good development, place pots in a sunny window or add additional grow lights.

Are Damiana plants susceptible to any pests or diseases?

Although daisies are generally resistant to pests and diseases, they can occasionally be impacted by powdery mildew, spider mites, or aphids. Regularly check plants, and use organic pest control techniques to quickly eradicate any infestations.

Is hydroponically grown Damiana possible?

Damiana can be grown hydroponically, however it could need certain tools and knowledge.

Strong growth and large harvests may be achieved by precisely controlling the fertilizer levels and growing environment with hydroponic systems.

How may Damiana plants be multiplied?

Seeds, stem cuttings, or division of existing plants can all be used to propagate Damiana. To propagate new plants, gather mature plant seeds and plant them in well-draining soil, or take stem cuttings and root them in a rooting media.

What is the typical lifetime of a plant called Damiana?

Perennial dahlia plants may survive for several years if given the right conditions. Proper trimming and upkeep can help Damiana plants live longer and develop more healthily.

Is it possible to cultivate Damiana with other plants or herbs?

In mixed beds or containers, damana can be planted with other herbs or plants. Herbs like sage, lavender, and rosemary are good companion plants because they draw beneficial insects to the garden and help keep pests away.

Addressing Concerns about Damiana's Aphrodisiac Effects

Is Damiana an aphrodisiac?

The traditional medical and folkloric uses of Damiana as an aphrodisiac date back many years. Although there is no scientific proof to back up Damiana's aphrodisiac properties, many individuals think it can increase libido and sexual excitement.

Does Damiana have any negative consequences when used as an aphrodisiac?

When used as directed, most people consider Damiana to be safe. However, some people could have adverse consequences including headaches, allergic reactions, or upset stomachs. Damiana must be used sensibly and sparingly to reduce the possibility of negative side effects.

Is it possible to treat sexual dysfunction with Damiana?

Damiana is used by some people as a natural treatment for sexual dysfunction, such as poor libido and erectile dysfunction. Damiana may be beneficial for sexual health and energy, but additional studies are required to clarify whether or not it works for treating certain ailments.

Is it okay to use Damiana when nursing or pregnant?

Information on Damiana's safety during pregnancy and lactation is scarce. Damiana has long been used to promote reproductive health, but little research has been done on whether it is safe to take during pregnancy or breastfeeding. Damiana should not be taken by pregnant or nursing mothers unless specifically instructed by a healthcare professional.

Does Damiana combine well with other vitamins or medications?

Certain drugs, such as sedatives, diabetic medications, and anticoagulants, may interact with Damiana. Before using Damiana, it is essential to speak with a licensed healthcare professional if you are taking any drugs or supplements to prevent any potential interactions.

What is the best way to prepare and ingest Damiana to get its aphrodisiac effects?

There are several ways to ingest Damiana, such as teas, tinctures, pills, or dried leaves. Damiana can be frequently ingested as a tincture or tea to get its possible aphrodisiac benefits. As needed, progressively raise the dosage while monitoring your body's reaction. Start with a modest amount.

Are there any situations when Damiana shouldn't be used as an aphrodisiac?

Before taking Damiana as an aphrodisiac, anyone with underlying medical disorders such as diabetes, cardiovascular disease, or hormone-sensitive malignancies should exercise caution and speak with a healthcare professional. In certain people, Damiana may worsen pre-existing medical issues or interfere with certain drugs.

CONCLUSION

We wish you well on your adventure with Damiana and encourage you to embrace innovation, experimentation, and an exploratory attitude. There are countless uses for damana in food, medicine, and aphrodisiacs, and there's always something new to learn.

Accept Diversity: Discover the wide range of Damiana cultivars and varietals, each with its distinct smells, scents, and qualities. Play around with different kinds to broaden your taste and improve your recipes.

Develop Curiosity: As you learn about Damiana's many facets, maintain an open mind and a curious disposition. Let your curiosity lead the way whether you're exploring the plant's therapeutic qualities, trying out new recipes, or improving cultivating methods.

Share Your Knowledge: Talk to others who are as passionate about Damiana as you are about your experiences and thoughts. Encourage a feeling of community and cooperation among enthusiasts through social media, community gardens, and online forums.

Celebrate Tradition: Pay tribute to Damiana's rich cultural past and its enduring customs in cooking, herbal medicine, and love rites. Honor the memory of people who have loved Damiana for many years and work to preserve its heritage even now.

Practice Sustainability: Grow Damiana using sustainable practices and with consideration for the environment. Encourage local farmers and groups that are committed to protecting Damiana's natural environment and encouraging moral farming methods.

Remain Curious: Remain aware of the most recent findings, patterns, and advancements in the production and application of damana. Continue to educate yourself on the best practices for responsible and safe usage, and be on the lookout for any possible hazards.

Damiana concludes by inviting us to go on a voyage of inquiry, learning, and kinship—to the environment, customs, and one another. May the endless potential of Damiana bring you happiness, inspiration, and contentment as you grow and experiment with it. Allow Damiana to accompany you on your journey to complete well-being, vigor, and intimacy—whether in the kitchen, the garden, or the bedroom.